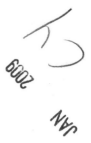
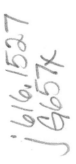

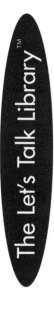

The Let's Talk Library™

Let's Talk About
Sickle Cell Anemia

Melanie Apel Gordon

The Rosen Publishing Group's
PowerKids Press™
New York

For Nancy Whisler and Michele Ottenfeld — Our circle is complete. Love, Melanie

Published in 2000 by The Rosen Publishing Group, Inc.
29 East 21st Street, New York, NY 10010

First Edition

Book Design: Erin McKenna

Photo Credits and Photo Illustrations: pp. 4, 12, 15, 20 by Les Mills; p. 7 © Robert Becker, Ph.D./Custom Medical; p. 8 © Custom Medical; p. 11 by Donna Scholl; p. 16 © Science Photo Library/Custom Medical; p. 19 © Science Photo Library/Custom Medical, (inset) © Custom Medical.

Gordon, Melanie Apel.
  Let's talk about sickle cell anemia / by Melanie Apel Gordon.
      p.   cm. — (The let's talk library)
  Summary: A simple introduction to sickle cell anemia, describing its symptoms, its effects on the body, and how to cope with this disease.
  Includes index.
  ISBN 0-8239-5417-X
  1. Sickle cell anemia—Juvenile literature. [1. Sickle cell anemia. 2. Diseases.] I. Title. II. Series.
  RC641.7.S5G67   1999
  616.1'527—dc21
                                                                                    98-39855
                                                                                          CIP
                                                                                          AC

Manufactured in the United States of America

Contents

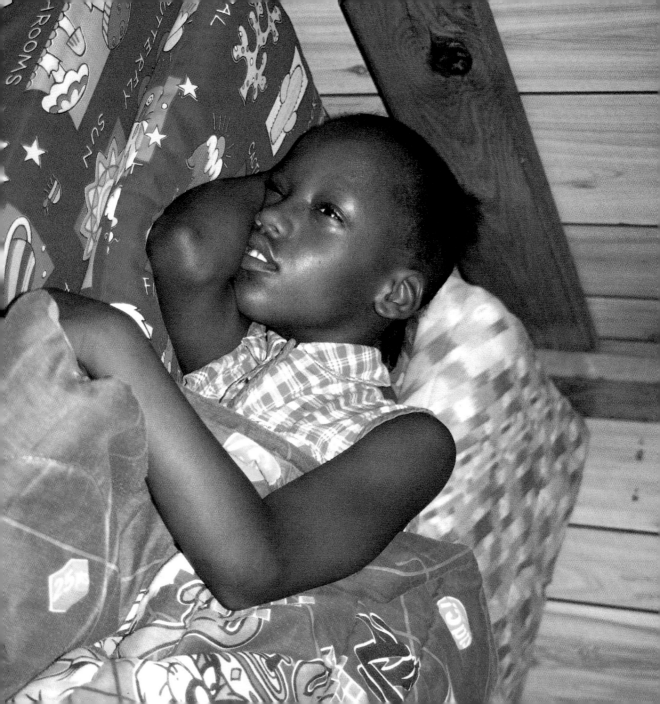

Jodie

Jodie looks out her bedroom window. She sees her friends playing outside. Jodie wants to go outside and play, too, but her legs hurt very badly. She has to stay in bed and drink lots of fluids and take medicine to help the pain go away. When Jodie feels better she can go outside and play with her friends. Jodie has **sickle cell anemia**. Right now she is having a sickle cell **crisis**.

▼ Sickle cell anemia crises don't happen all the time. But when they do happen they aren't much fun.

Hemoglobin

Hemoglobin is a **protein** in your red blood cells that gives your blood its red color. Hemoglobin's job is to carry **oxygen** from your lungs to the cells in the rest of your body. Red blood cells with normal hemoglobin are soft and flexible. They are shaped like doughnuts and can easily squeeze through your blood vessels to get the oxygen to where it needs to go. After hemoglobin drops off the oxygen, your red blood cells are still shaped like doughnuts and are ready to pick up more oxygen.

This is what healthy red blood cells look like. ▶

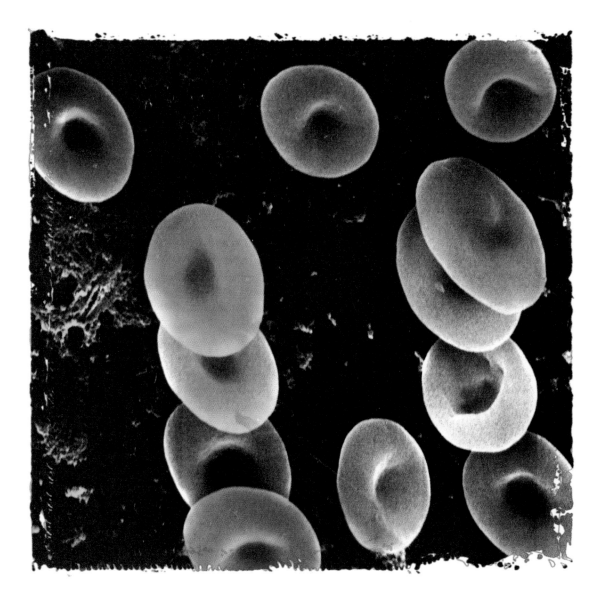

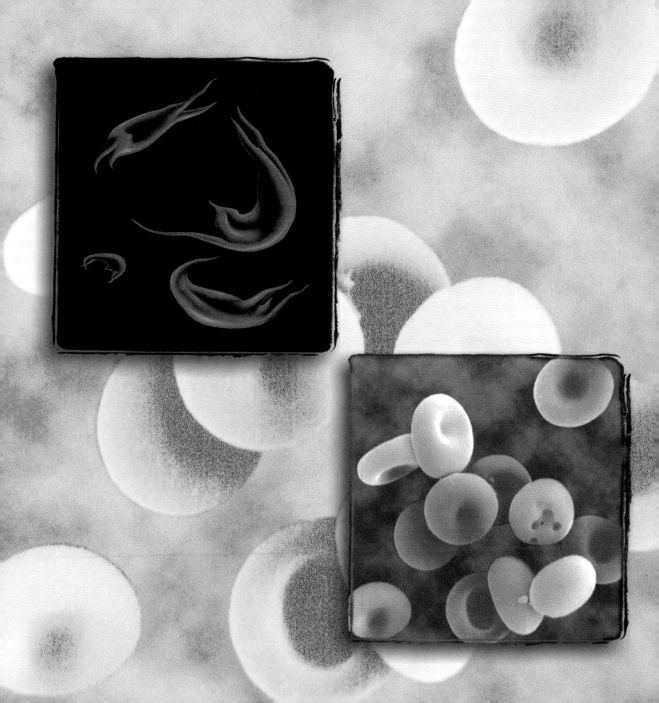

Sickled Cells

People who have sickle cell anemia have different hemoglobin. It is called hemoglobin S. After hemoglobin S drops off oxygen, it causes the red blood cell to change shape. The cell becomes crescent-shaped, kind of like the moon. These cells are rough and hard. They can't move through blood vessels very easily. Sometimes they get stuck, and then they can't deliver oxygen. If oxygen can't get to your cells you may feel pain in your arms, legs, back, chest, or stomach. This is called sickle cell crisis. A crisis can happen at any time.

▼ The top picture shows healthy red blood cells. The bottom picture shows sickled red blood cells.

Who Has Sickle Cell Anemia?

Most people who have sickle cell anemia are African or African American. Some people who are Greek, Spanish, Indian, Italian, or from the Caribbean Islands have it too. More than 60,000 people in the United States have sickle cell anemia. This disease is not **contagious**. That means that you can't catch it from someone who has it. People who have sickle cell anemia are born with it.

You can't tell if people have sickle cell anemia just by looking at them. ▶

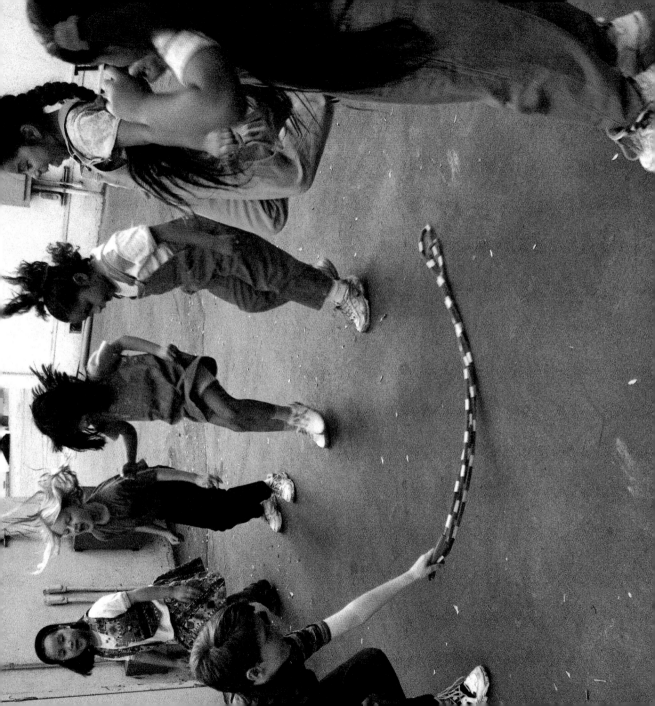

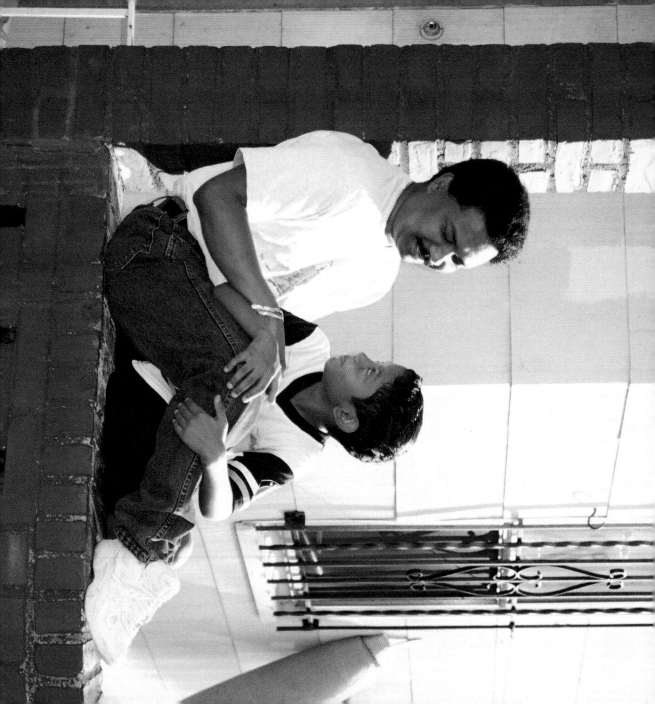

Heredity

Sickle cell anemia is **hereditary**. That means that it gets passed down from your parents to you. To get sickle cell anemia, you have to **inherit** two **genes** for sickle cell anemia, one from each parent. If you inherit only one gene, or if only one of your parents has the gene, then you won't get sickle cell anemia. But you will have **sickle cell trait**. This won't make you sick. But you will be a **carrier**. This means that even though you do not have sickle cell anemia, you can still pass the gene on to your children.

▶ You get many traits from your parents. Hair color, eye color, and right- or left-handedness all come from your parents' genes.

Sickle Cell Trait

About 2.5 million people in the United States carry the sickle cell gene in their bodies. People who have sickle cell trait do not have **symptoms** of sickle cell anemia. This is because only about 30 percent of their red blood cells are sickled. That's not enough to make them sick. But people who have sickle cell trait can pass it on to their children. And people who have sickle cell trait might have a problem if they fly in an airplane because there isn't as much oxygen way up high in the sky.

People who have sickle cell trait usually don't suffer from crises the way people with sickle cell anemia do. ▶

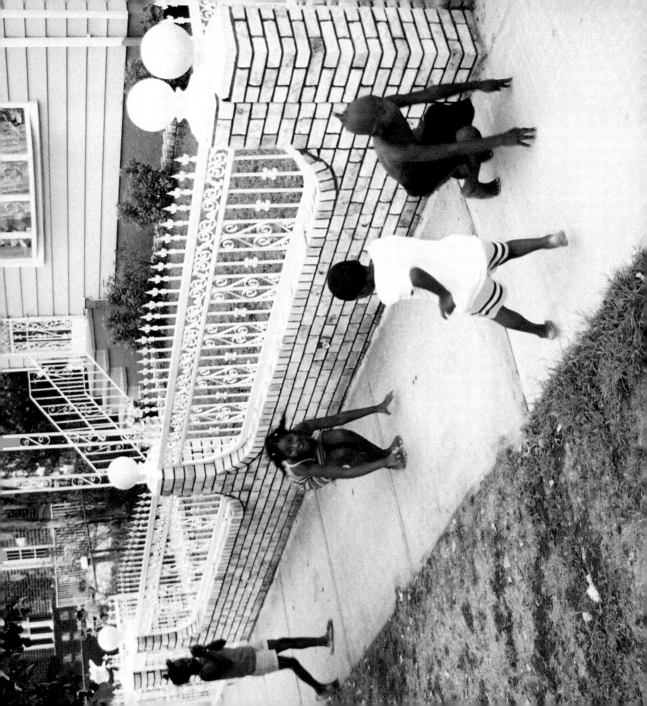

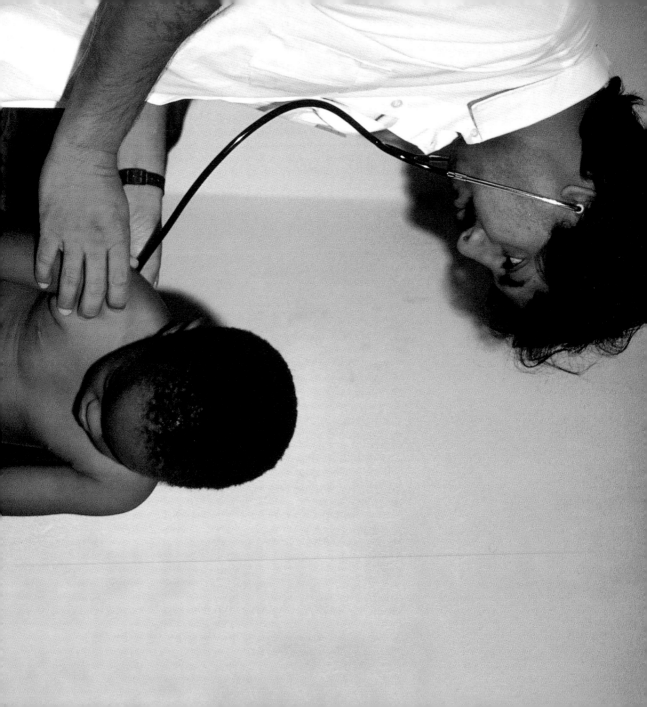

Symptoms

When parts of your body do not get enough oxygen you will feel the symptoms of sickle cell anemia. Some of the symptoms of sickle cell anemia are:

- pain in the arms, legs, stomach, and back
- swollen hands and feet
- sores on your legs that heal very slowly
- growing more slowly than other kids
- getting sick more often than other kids do

If you have all or most of these symptoms your doctor can test your blood to see if you have sickle cell anemia.

▼ Your doctor can test you for sickle cell anemia and give you medicine if you have a crisis.

Where Did It Come From?

Sickle cell anemia has been around for thousands of years. But it was first studied and named in 1904. Sickle cell anemia started in Africa. And when people who had the sickle cell gene left Africa, they brought hemoglobin S with them. Now it is in all parts of the world. Scientists think that hemoglobin S may protect people from a disease called **malaria.** Malaria is a serious disease that is common in very warm places like Africa. And even though hemoglobin S causes a painful disease, it also helps protect people from a different disease.

Malaria is spread by the anopheles mosquito. If you have hemoglobin S, you are protected from the disease. ▼

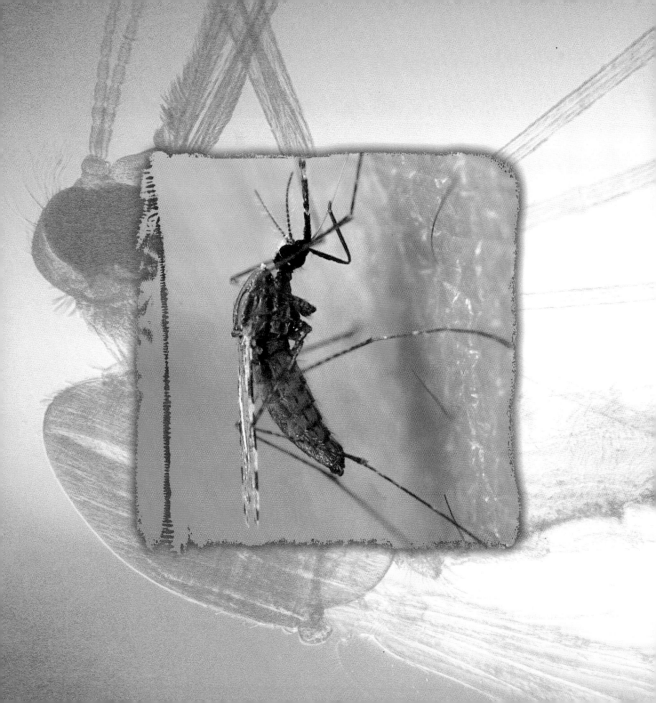

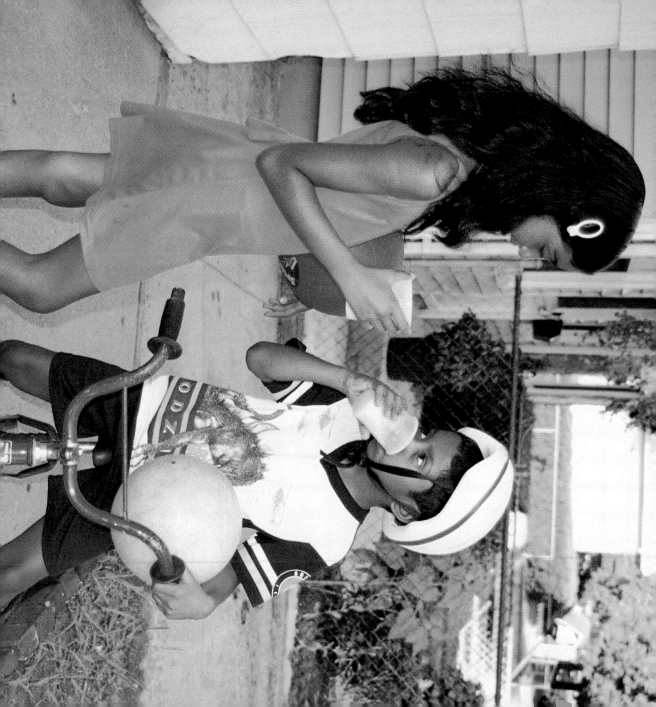

Treatment

There is no cure for sickle cell anemia. But you can take care of its symptoms. Your doctor will tell you to drink lots of fluids and take pain medicine when you are in crisis. Sometimes, if your crisis is very bad, you may have to go to the hospital. At the hospital you may be given extra oxygen, blood **transfusions**, or **IV** fluids to help you feel better.

▶ Drinking lots of fluids, especially after exercise, helps keep people with sickle cell anemia from having a crisis.

Taking Care of Yourself Every Day

If you have sickle cell anemia you will have a pain crisis now and then. You may even have to go to the hospital sometimes. But you can do your best to help your body get enough oxygen by drinking lots of fluids, resting after exercising, avoiding alcohol and cigarettes, and not flying in airplanes. If you do all of these things, you will keep your body healthy and be able to do many of the things that you enjoy.

Glossary

carrier (KAR-eer) A person whose cells carry a specific gene.

contagious (kun-TAY-jus) When a sickness can be passed from one person to another.

crisis (CRY-sis) When sickle cell anemia causes severe pain.

gene (JEEN) A tiny part of your cells that you get from your parents.

hemoglobin (HEE-muh-gloh-bin) A protein in your red blood cells that carries oxygen from your lungs to the cells in the rest of your body.

hereditary (huh-REH-dih-ter-ee) Passed down from your parents to you.

inherit (in-HER-it) To get something from your parents.

IV (EYE VEE) A tube that allows medicine and fluids to flow directly into your body—usually through your arm.

malaria (muh-LARE-ee-uh) A serious disease common in very warm places, such as Africa.

oxygen (AHK-sih-jin) A gas present in air that is necessary for people and animals to breathe.

protein (PROH-teen) An important substance inside the cells of people, plants, and animals.

sickle cell anemia (SIH-kul SELL uh-NEE-mee-uh) A hereditary disease that causes abnormal hemoglobin and sickle-shaped red blood cells.

sickle cell trait (SIH-kul SELL TRAYT) When a person has only one gene for sickle cell anemia.

symptom (SIMP-tum) Something you feel that lets you know you are sick.

transfusion (tranz-FYOO-zhun) The transferring of blood from someone else into your body.

Index